YOGA
Simple Stretches and Postures
for the Less Able

YOGA
Simple Stretches and Postures
for the Less Able

Eileen Oliver

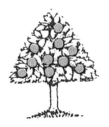

THE ERSKINE PRESS

2013

YOGA
Simple Stretches and Postures
for the Less Able

First published in 2013 by The Erskine Press,
The White House, Eccles, Norwich, NR16 2PB
WWW.ERSKINE-PRESS.COM

ISBN 978 1 85297115 1
The moral right of the author has been asserted

A CIP catalogue record is available from the British Library

Designed and produced by *jackafrika Associates*
Printed and bound in Great Britain by
Barkers Print & Design Limited

CONTENTS

Yoga is not competitive nor is it about force or strain.
Do not struggle to achieve a position
that your body is not ready for.
It will tell you when it is.

YOGA FOR THE LESS ABLE

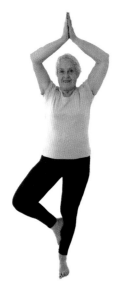

I have reached my three score years and ten, have practiced Yoga for 38 years and of those have been a teacher for ten. I have always had a very stiff, inflexible body and I needed to work very hard to keep my mobility and flexibility alive and well. Recently, I have had a burning desire to write a book for people of my age who would like to try Yoga but who perhaps feel they are too old and stiff to have a go. I would like to inspire these people, to tell them it's never too late. They may not be the Yogi of the year but they might just be able to improve on their strength, balance and flexibility.

It is very important to maintain what you have, rather than to allow your body and mind to go slowly downhill. Some gentle practice could lower blood pressure and help keep the heart strong. We cannot avoid old age but we can certainly keep it at the gate for a little longer by helping ourselves in this way.

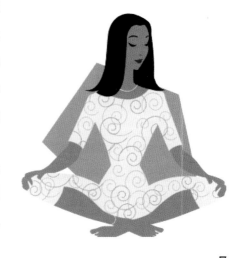

If you decide to try Yoga you need to be aware that it will change your whole outlook on life, and for the better. If you don't want this to happen, don't practice Yoga. One aspect of practicing Yoga is that with conscientious practice, mindfulness and living in the moment become a habit – which is extremely helpful in older age, especially if you have reached the stage of wandering into a room or going upstairs and then asking yourself 'What have I come here for?' It also helps to alleviate worry and to calm the nerves, which seems to become more of a problem when accompanied by a fear of old age and what the future holds.

Yoga, if it has been modified to suit the needs and capabilities of the individual student, is for everyone. Even if the student only learns to breathe correctly, the time has been well spent. So many benefits can be gained from the gentle and realistic practice of breathing (*pranayama*), from stretching and exercise (*asana*), and from relaxation and contemplation (using music or an object to aid the focusing of the mind), all of which, hopefully, will lead on to meditation. One doesn't have to be a Sanskrit expert or travel to a guru in India in order to become knowledgeable and to be an able practitioner of Yoga.

Consistent weekly or, preferably, daily practice will eventually lead to a healthier body, a sharper mind and a contentment that is difficult to describe. For best results I suggest you join a suitable class and then try to cultivate the habit of a little regular practice. There is no better way than to have guidance from a teacher.

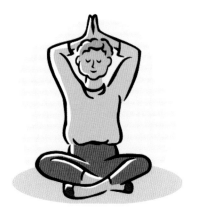

Once the feeling of well-being kicks in, you will automatically start to take more care of your body by watching the foods you eat, (no longer eating junk food), not smoking, lowering alcohol consumption and getting enough sleep. You may also feel a need to spend time alone in peaceful, uplifting surroundings, mixing with like-minded people and reading helpful uplifting literature to help you on your journey to a better life.

Eileen Oliver
S.R.N. O.N.C.
B.W.Y. Teacher Trained

Just Breathe!

1
ABOUT YOGA

What is Yoga?

Yoga translated means union, and if practiced mindfully will bring perfect harmony of body, mind and spirit and a union of the little self with the greater self; union of the soul with its infinite source, God or who ever we recognize as our creator.'

The British Wheel of Yoga handout

Sri Swami Sivanavanada in his booklet 'The Science of Yoga' says: 'Yoga brings a message of hope to the forlorn, joy to the depressed, knowledge to the ignorant, and strength to the weak. It is the secret master-key that unlocks the realm of Elysian bliss and deep, abiding peace.'

Yoga is life. It is a method which overhauls all aspects of the human personality. It is a system of integral education, education not only of the body and the mind or the intellect, but also of the inner spirit. Yoga shows you the marvellous method of rising from evil to good, and from goodness to holiness and then to eternal divine splendour. Yoga is the art of right living. The Yogi who has learned the art of right living is happy, harmonious, peaceful and free from tension. Yoga is a science perfected by seers in India, not merely of India, but of humanity as a whole. It is an exact science, a perfect, practical system of self-culture.

The British Wheel of Yoga handout

A Way of Life

Yoga does not require turning away from life – it demands transformation and spiritualisation of life. Yoga is primarily a way of life, not something which is divorced from life. Yoga is not forsaking an action, but is an efficient performance in the right spirit. Yoga is not running away from home and human habitation, but a process of moulding one's attitude to home and society with a new understanding.

Yoga Sutras of Patanjali

Yoga is Universal

Yoga is for all and is universal; it is not a sectarian affair, but a way to God and not a creed. The practice of Yoga is not opposed to any religion or any sacred church. It is purely spiritual and universal and does not contradict anyone's sincere faith. Yoga is not a religion, but an aid to the practice of the basic spiritual truths in all religions. It can be practiced by Christians or a Buddhist, a Parsee, Mohammedans, a Sufi or an atheist. To be a Yogi means to abide continuously in God and to live at peace with men. Yoga is union with God, union with all. God dwells in all.

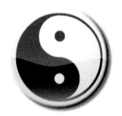

The British Wheel of Yoga handout

Yoga takes you into the present moment, the only place where life exists.

DIET

I do not wish to talk too much about diet as there is an excess of literature on healthy eating. The body is a temple for the soul: not only does it need exercise but it needs to be nourished with good wholesome food (*Satvic*), which is simple fresh produce low in additives, artificial colouring, sugar and salt. Take care to avoid addictive substances and drink plenty of water. Balance is the object. Raw food is more beneficial than cooked but steaming is ideal.

A vegetarian diet is highly conducive to clear thinking and divine contemplation. It is said to render the intellect keen, subtle and sharp. Potatoes, rice, grains, pulses, tomatoes, green beans, radishes, carrots, cucumber, spinach and green leafy vegetables and fresh fruit are all good and pure and give greater vitality than animal foods. Avoid too many condiments, spices, tea, coffee and alcohol and foods that are very rich in starch, sugar and fats. A simple diet that avoids unnecessary foods will help to relieve strain on the liver and kidneys. Leave the table with the feeling that you could have eaten a little more.

Many Yogis choose to be vegetarian but this is not essential. Those who eat meat try to honour the animal that gave its life by not being wasteful, not cooking and eating too much and maybe eating meat only once or twice a week. Meat is said to spoil the health, excite passion and make the mind restless. Eat only when hungry, masticate food well and drink plenty of water after meals, but not during because it dilutes the gastric juices.

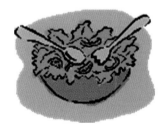

SOME YOGA TERMS AND THEIR MEANING

Hatha Yoga

Hatha Yoga is a practice that combines slow and gentle movements with breathing exercises to create a feeling of relaxation. The whole package is comprised of eight 'limbs' that, when practised carefully and mindfully, will lead to a happiness and contentment within, rather than the expectation of finding such happiness in a material lifestyle of possessions and money. It also raises a spiritual awareness, hence the union of mind, body and spirit. Students learn an awareness of their body/energy/space/*prana* (life force) and spirit. A positive outlook, the enjoyment of silence and living in the moment, become more evident to the person and to the observer.

The 'eight limbs' of Hatha Yoga

1) *Yamas* – disciplines that concern the way we treat our environment and the people around us: for example not harming anyone or anything; truthfulness; not stealing.

2) *Nyamas*- disciplines that concern the way we look after ourselves – cleanliness (in our body and our home); contentedness; self discipline (eating good wholesome food, having enough rest and sleep, not smoking and drinking to excess etc).

3) *Asana* – learning to hold poses in stillness, with a calm and steady breath, to encourage mental equilibrium. The 'Lotus Position' is possibly the most well-known *asana*. For advanced students only, it is always associated with *Hatha Yoga*.

4) *Pranayama* – breath control.

5) *Pratyahara* – the withdrawal of the senses. The mind naturally turns inwards during Yoga practice, which brings the outward direction of the senses – sight, hearing, taste, smell and touch – *under control.*

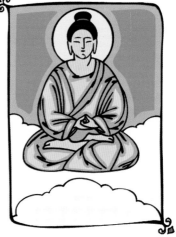

6) *Dharana* – concentration; mental focus achieved through posture together with breath awareness and control.

7) *Dhyana* – meditation; developing the practice of enjoying quiet andcontrolled focus of thought.

8) *Samadhi* – enlightenment or self-realisation; bliss.

Asana

'*Asana* is a comfortable and steady pose' (Yoga Sutras of Patanjali). *Asana* is the Sanskrit term for seated posture but generally, in Western Hatha Yoga, it just means 'posture'.

The British Wheel of Yoga handout

The purpose of *asana* is to build a firm, strong and supple body. The focus, concentration and awareness needed in good practice in turn trains the mind to be more focused and aware, help-ing memory performance in everyday life. The aim for the practitioner is to eventually meditate without distraction as our bodies will be strong and flexible enough to sit for long periods. The purpose of Yoga is to develop the union of mind, body and soul through practice, and *asana* is the very first step on this journey.

Although meditation sessions often use a seated *asana* as a comfortable position in which to practice, general Hatha Yoga classes offer postures for other reasons. For example, as classic Yoga texts say:

♦ To remain physically and mentally steady, calm, quiet and comfortable;

♦ To allow practitioners to develop a stable foundation from which to explore deeper Yoga practices.

By regularly practicing *asana* you may notice the following:

♦ An increased feeling of vitality and strength;

♦ A more balanced feeling – light and joyful, with increasing awareness;

♦ A better ability to relax, concentrate and meditate;

♦ A more effective digestion and improved general body and muscle tone.

The ancient teachings use a beautiful story to illustrate the unfolding of the spiritual nature of humans. The symbolic Lotus flower grows in the murky swamps. It sends roots down into the mud to hold it firm in the unpredictable nature of the water, and sends a flowering stem up towards the light, opening its petals to embrace the warmth and life force of the sun.

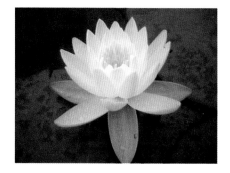

Prana

If you take up the practice of Yoga seriously you will come across *prana*. A Sanskrit word, *prana* translates into English as breath or life force; the all-pervading vital energy which enters the body on conception, sustains us through life and departs at death. Swami Muktibodhananda from the Bihar School of Yoga says, '*prana* is the tangible manifestation of the higher self'- it is God within us. Without *prana* there is no life. It enters the body on the breath but is separate from the gases of the air. It can be experienced more acutely at the sea-side or in the mountains.

Pranayama

Prana means 'breath', *ayama* means to lengthen/expand/extend, so the practice increases the *prana* in the body by improving, lengthening and expanding the breath; hence *pranayama*.

Part of the Yoga practice is concerned with breathing, because the breath and mind are very closely connected. If the breath is calm the mind will also be calm, so by controlling one, the other is also under control. Focusing on the breath is an excellent way to calm the mind. This is why the Yogi considers the practice of *pranayama* to be so important.

Simple forms of *pranayama* can be practiced by most people without any harm. More advanced practice with breath retention needs the guidance of a tutor. You should use common sense if you suffer from a heart or lung condition, high blood pressure, if you are pregnant or generally feeling unwell. It is up to you to be responsible for your own body. If it feels uncomfortable or if you are struggling then ease back and take it more gently.

USEFUL TIPS AND CAUTIONS

a) In any programme of exercise there is a possibility of injury, especially so with an older body or when you have not exercised for some time. This should not, however, stop you from trying. Begin gently and avoid strain and over-zealousness.

b) If you have a history of heart disease, high blood pressure, chronic arthritis or some other injury or serious condition, or if you are on strong medication, consult your doctor about what you plan to do.

c) Do not exercise if you have just drunk alcohol as it could impair judgment.

d) Wait for 1½-2hrs after a heavy meal before exercising or meditating.

e) Try to exercise at the same time every day.

f) Read the instructions for each posture carefully.

g) If necessary, use a chair or the wall for support.

h) Try to exercise in a warm place. A bath or shower beforehand can help to loosen you up.

i) Keep movement and breathing slow and smooth to enable you to stop if necessary.

j) It is better to do a few exercises each day rather than many once a week.

k) Wear comfortable clothing, leave your feet bare and exercise on a non-slip floor. If you can do floor exercises it is nice to have a non-slip Yoga mat. You may also need a block, a strap and a cushion and blanket for relaxation.

l) Learn the movements of postures before attempting to incorporate the breathing.

m) After a hip replacement follow any special advice given by the consultant in charge of the operation, (for example NOT CROSSING LEGS) and then work within your capabilities and strength. The same applies to knee replacements. Kneeling will be a problem which can sometimes be overcome by using a 2″ thick block or thick padding under the leg, avoiding the knee joint. Otherwise adapt exercises and either stand or use a chair.

n) If you are not confident and need help, practice with a friend or family member.

<u>CHAKRAS</u>

Chakra is a Sanskrit word which means 'wheel' or 'revolving disc' – a vortex of energy. Our bodies have an electro-magnetic field, seen by many as the 'aura', which is made up of the energy which vibrates on different frequencies and manifests itself as the colours of the rainbow.

When the *chakras* are whirling and spinning freely the system is balanced. When a *chakra* is blocked then our physical and mental well-being can be affected.

The *chakras* – these wheels – are energy centres and there are seven main ones referred to in Yoga. They are aligned along the spinal column and connected to us on several different levels: physical, mental, emotional and spiritual. The lotus flower is often used to symbolise the *chakras*.

1st Chakra (MULADHARA) A lotus with 4 petals (the base *chakra*).

Meaning: 'The root of our support' – the base *chakra*

Location: Perineum at the base of the spine

Colour: Red

Element: Earth

Governs: The kidneys, adrenal glands, pelvis, hips, knees, lower back, sciatic nerve and bowel movements.

2nd Chakra (SVADISTHANA) – A six petal lotus.

Meaning: 'Your own dwelling place' – commonly known as the sexual centre

Location: Between the genitals and navel

Colour: Orange

Element: Water

Governs: Genitalia, reproductive organs, bladder and prostate.

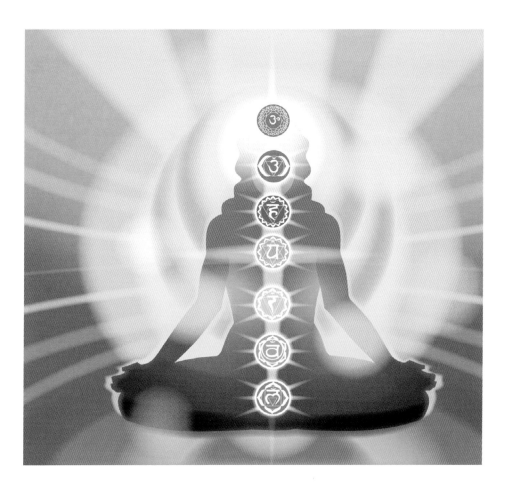

(from bottom to top)

1. Muladhara: the 1st—root— chakra

2. Svadisthana: the 2nd—sacral— chakra

3. Manipura: the 3rd—solar plexus—chakra

4. Anahata: the 4th—heart—chakra

5. Vishuddha: the 5th—throat—chakra

6. Ajna: the 6th—third eye—chakra

7. Sahasrara: the 7th—crown—chakra

3rd Chakra (MANIPURA) – A lotus with ten petals.

Meaning: 'Dwelling place of jewels' – commonly known as the power centre

Location: At the solar plexus

Colour: Yellow

Element: Fire

Governs: The spleen, liver, gall bladder, stomach and pancreas.

4th Chakra (ANAHATA) – A lotus with twelve petals.

Meaning: 'That which is ever new' – commonly known as the heart centre

Location: At the centre of the chest

Colour: Green

Element: Air

Governs: The physical heart, lungs and thymus gland.

5th Chakra (VISHUDDHA) – A lotus with sixteen petals.

Meaning: 'Purest of the pure' – known as the throat chakra

Location: The throat

Colour: Blue

Element: Ether or space

Governs: The vocal chords, thyroid, voice and hearing.

6th Chakra (AJNA) – A lotus with two petals.

Meaning: 'Command' – commonly known as the third eye

Location: The centre of the forehead between

              the eye brows

Colour: Indigo

Element: Light

Governs: The pituitary gland.

7th Chakra (SAHASRARA) – The 1000 petal lotus.

Meaning: 'A 1000 petal lotus'

Location: At the crown of the head

Colour: Violet, white or gold

Governs: The pineal gland.

There are postures that have a particular benefit for each *chakra* but no posture works on only one *chakra* at a time. Each posture will affect more than one.

Kundalini

Kundalini is symbolically referred to as the coiled serpent that sits at the base of the spine in the base *chakra*. As we develop awareness of our subtle energy and we become more aware of our creator in our lives, this energy is said to rise up an invisible channel just in front of the spinal column, passing through each *chakra* until it

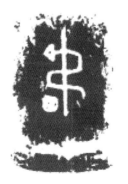

reaches the crown. The more centred and balanced we become, the higher it goes. When the *kundalini* reaches the crown *chakra* it is said that *samadhi* or spiritual enlightenment is reached and the Yogi attains liberation and divine wealth.

2
BREATH AWARENESS

The importance of the breath

It is important that when we start practicing the postures we also pay attention to the breath, and become aware of the part it plays in each movement. For example, through necessity, we tend to inhale on opening up and exhale on a folding movement. It is difficult to breathe in when the body is folded forwards. Being mindful of the breath helps us to focus and develop concentration. It is also important not to hold the breath and build up tension because the body does not work well when it is tense. The breath needs to flow and keep the blood oxygenated to give the body the energy with which to work.

    Firstly, it's a good idea to explore the regions of the chest and the movement of the rib cage with the diaphragm.

a)   Stand comfortably or sit on a chair, or on the floor using a block or kneeling device. The spine should be straight and the shoulders relaxed.

b)   Place your hands on the abdomen just below the ribs, breathe in and allow the abdomen to swell or expand. This is brought about by the diaphragm (a large dome shaped muscle which separates the lungs from the abdominal organs) flattening.

c) Now breathe out allowing the abdomen to contract and flatten. This is referred to as abdominal breathing.

d) Do this several times to get the feel of it.

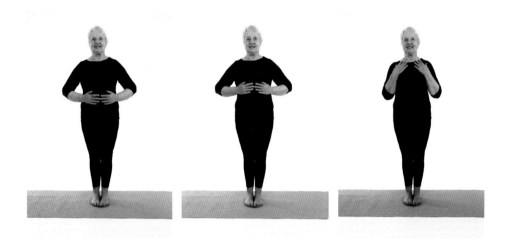

When comfortable with this practice move on to the rib cage.

a) Place your hands on the lower rib cage, breathe in and feel the ribs lift up and out. Breathe out and feel the rib cage drop down and in. Practice this for a few breaths.

b) Place your hands on the ribs just below the armpits. Breathe in and try to isolate some movement in this area.

c) Place your hands on the upper chest with finger tips touching the clavicle or collar bones. Breathe in and hopefully feel the lift in the rib cage.

d) Place your hands on the back and try to find some movement in this area. This can be done with a partner. Kneel on all fours or sit on a chair.

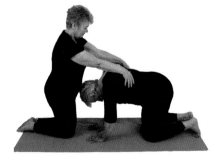

Your partner places their hands on the rib cage in order to feel the movement.

Having mastered the above it is time to try to put it all together.

e)   Breathe gently down into the abdomen and then allow the lungs to fill right to the top. Pause for a very brief second and breathe out steadily and slowly. As you practice make the 'out' breath longer than the 'in' breath. This technique is the basis of good breathing and should be practiced well before moving on to other, more complicated, exercises. This can be practiced standing, sitting or lying down.

A standing 'complete breath and stretching' warm up

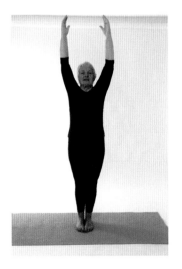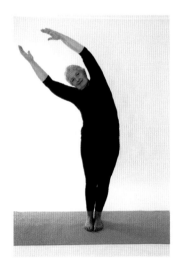

a)   Stand tall with your feet together.

b)   Breathing in, raise the arms above the head. Breathe out and stretch over to the side. Breathe in and come up to the centre. Breathe out and stretch to the other side. Breathe in and come back to the centre.

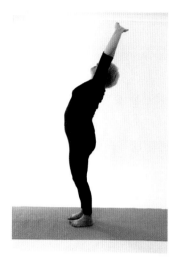 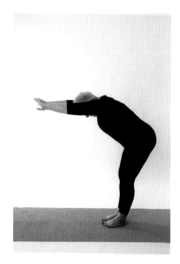

c)   Hold the breath and stretch up gently, or backwards if there are no problems with the neck or with giddiness.

d)   Breathe out, bending forwards (not too far). Breathe in, coming back to the centre, breathe out and lower the arms to the side.

Repeat this 2 or 3 times, starting with a different side each time.

3
WARM-UP PRACTICE
(SITTING OR KNEELING)

> **It is important to practice warm-up exercises to prepare the body for stronger posture work.**

Pavanmuktasana – a joint-freeing sequence by Mukunda Stiles which can be used as a daily practice .

Ankles – seated

a) Inhale, point the foot, curl the toes; exhale, draw the foot back, spread the toes.

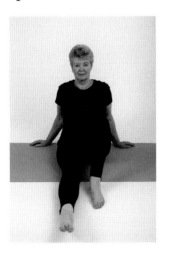 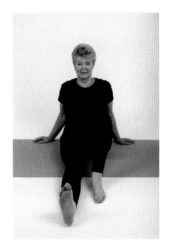

b) Inhale, turn the soles in towards each other; exhale, turn them out.

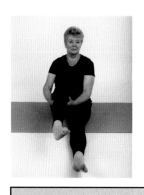

c) Holding a bent leg, circle the foot outwards. Then circle it inwards, and finally circle both feet.

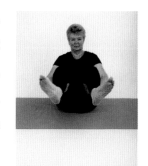

Practice these movements as slowly and positively as you can, getting as full a movement as possible. Do this several times to each side, trying to work with the breath, keeping a steady in and out breath with each hug in.

Knees & hips

Seated, either on a chair or on the floor, inhale, extend the leg; exhale, bend and hug alternate knees to the chest.

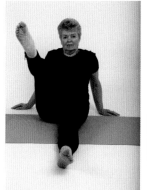

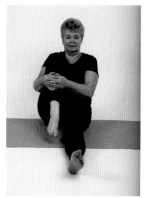

Hips

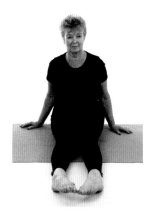

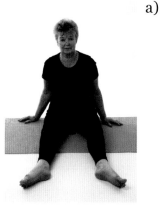

a) Seated with the legs straight, a little more than hip width apart, inhale, turn the legs outward; exhale, turn the legs inward.

30

b) Inhale, circle one knee up and out; exhale, circle it down and in, making the movement as wide and as open as possible. Reverse the direction and then work with the other knee.

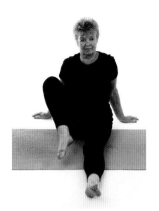

c) Again sitting on the floor, bend the

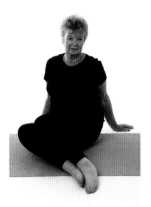 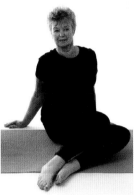

knees and lean back on the hands. Inhale, exhale and roll the knees to the side; inhale and bring the legs up to the centre. Exhale and roll to the other side.

Wrists

Kneeling or seated, with the palms facing down, inhale, curl the hands into a fist, exhale, extend and stretch the fingers as wide as possible. See more hand exercises in Chapter 5.

Elbows

Still kneeling or seated, inhale, extend the arms; exhale, flex or bend the elbows.

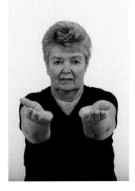 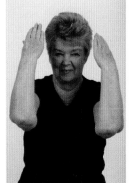

Shoulder rotation

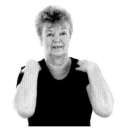

Still kneeling or seated, bring the fingers to the shoulders, inhale; take the elbows back and wide; exhale_and bring the elbows forward, making as large a circle as possible. Do this several_times, then rotate the shoulders in the opposite direction.

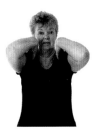 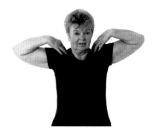 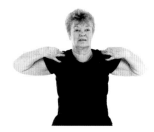

Side stretch

Sit up really straight in a cross-legged position or with the legs out in front of you. Relax the shoulders. Inhale and raise the arms to shoulder height. As you exhale place one hand on the floor and stretch the other up and over the head. Hold for a moment or two, inhale and come back to the centre. Stretch up again, exhale and stretch to the opposite side in the same manner.

Release the legs if necessary, then reposition with crossed or straight legs. This could also be done sitting on a chair, stretching as far as possible.

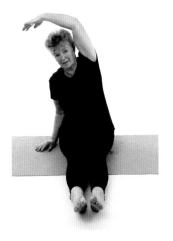 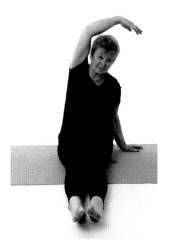

Seated twist

Stretch and lift the body up straight; inhale and take the left arm across to the outside of the opposite thigh. Exhale, raise the right arm, twist the body round to

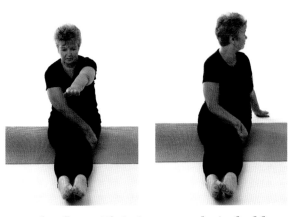

look behind, taking the arm to the floor. If sitting on a chair, hold on to the opposite back of the chair with the right hand. This will help to gain extra stretch. Hold for a moment or two and release. Repeat to the other side.

Cat stretch in a sitting position

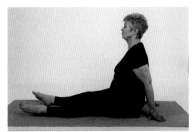

Sit up straight and take the arms a little way behind the body, touching the floor (or the back of the chair if using one). Inhale, then on the out-breath stretch and arch the body forward, flexing the spine. Hold for a moment or two, inhale and on the out- breath take the body into a gentle backward bend, extending the spine. Hold and return to the centre. Repeat several times in a continuous movement. Relax and allow the breath to settle. Remember to relax the neck and shoulders on the forward bend.

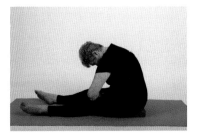

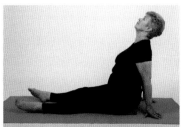

33

Neck – (seated)

Inhale, take the chin up and forward; exhale, take the chin down. Inhale to the centre; exhale and take the ear to the shoulder; inhale and take the head back to the centre. Repeat on the other side.

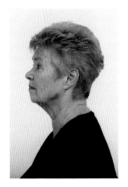 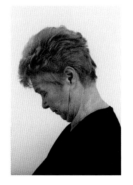 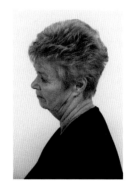

Inhale to the centre; exhale, turn the head from side to side keeping the chin level. Exhale and return to the centre.

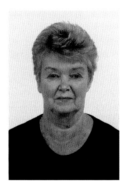 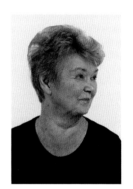

How to get up from the floor

If you have not done these exercises before and do not feel comfortable, don't attempt them unless you are in a class situation or have a companion who could help you up in an emergency.

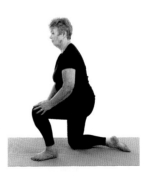

If you have the strength and confidence to do without a chair, then come on to your knees

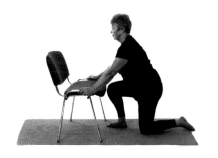 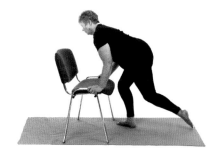

and kneeling up, place one foot on the floor in front of you. With your hands on your bent knee, push up gracefully. Alternatively, work close to a wall, using it or a chair to steady yourself.

The Yoga pose that you avoid the most,
you need the most.

4
WARM-UP PRACTICE
(LYING)

Basic stretch

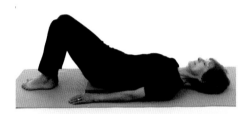

Lie on the floor in semi-supine (on your back with the knees bent). Inhale; take the arms up and over the head to touch the floor if possible. Exhale and return the arms to the side of the body. Repeat a few times, synchronizing the breath with the movement.

Then continue: inhale, take the arms over the head. Exhale, lower the arms and bring the right knee to the chest and hug in. Then return the leg to the floor. Inhale, raise the arms again but this time changing legs and hugging the left knee to the

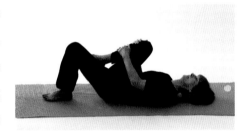

chest. Repeat three times.

Keeping the arm movement the same, now hug both legs to the chest on exhalation. Repeat three times.

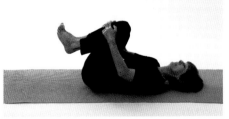

Continue the arm and leg movements, again hugging both legs to the chest while bringing the forehead towards the knees – if you are comfortable doing so. Relax back to semi-supine.

Leg stretch with strap

Place a strap or belt around the ball of the foot and stretch the leg up to the ceiling, trying to straighten it. If this is easy then, using the strap, draw the leg towards the body as you inhale. Exhale to relax. Keep gently stretching and easing with the breath. Repeat with the other leg.

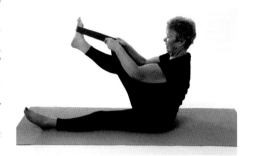

Leg stretch

Proceed with the next warm-up exercise, starting in semi-supine. Breathe in, raise both arms and a straight leg to the ceiling; then while breathing out, lower both arms and the leg to the floor. Repeat three times. Inhale, raise the arms and the other leg. Repeat three times.

Twist

Staying in semi-supine take the arms out to the side at shoulder level, keeping the legs tight together. Inhale, then exhale and lower the bent legs to the right side as far as they will go. Turn the head to the left. Inhale, tighten the abdominal

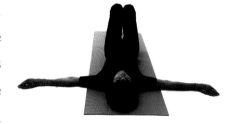

muscles and lift the knees to the centre. Exhale and lower the knees to the left, this time turning the head to the right. Inhale, tighten the abdominal muscles and lift the legs back to the centre. Repeat 3 times. Try to keep the shoulders firmly on the floor and allow gravity to encourage the knees down.

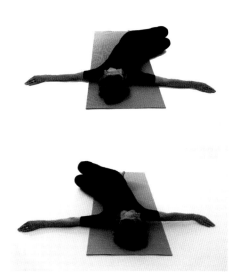

Rainbow twist

Another alternative twist is to lie on your side, knees slightly bent and both arms out straight in front at shoulder level. You may need

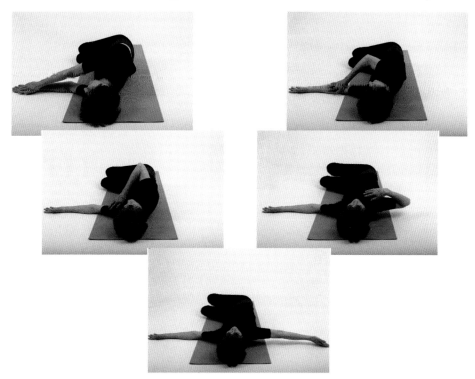

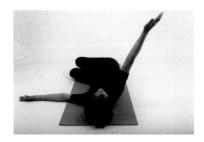 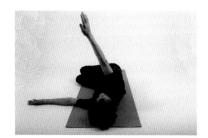

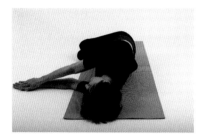

a block or folded blanket under your head. As you inhale slide the left hand along the arm and across the chest. As you exhale curl the arm down onto the floor behind. Keep this position for a few moments then on an inhalation lift the left arm, raising it towards the ceiling and lowering it to the original position as you exhale. Repeat three times. Go to the other side and repeat.

Cycling

Place the hands on the floor with a block under the pelvis. Peddle the legs in the air very positively, making the movement as big as possible. Do this several times then reverse the action. Relax in semi-supine.

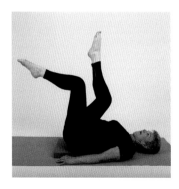 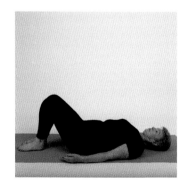

Open pose

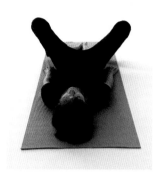

Lie in semi-supine. Bring the soles of the feet together and allow the knees to part, dropping outwards to the floor. You may need to place a pillow under your head and knees if the back arches too much and you cannot relax comfortably into the posture. Bring your hands together in prayer position – *namaste.*

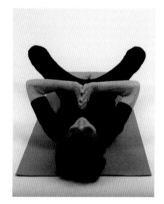

Breathe deeply several times and try to let the body relax into the posture. When ready to come out of the posture place a hand under each knee and lift the legs back to the centre. Straighten the legs.

Bridge

Lie in semi-supine with the legs hip-width apart and the feet firmly on the floor. Remove any padding from under the head. Relax the arms by the side of the body, flatten the back onto the floor and pull

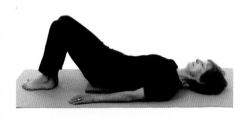

the navel to the spine. As you inhale, slowly curl the spine up off the floor to raise the whole body a few inches, pushing the pubic bone to the ceiling.

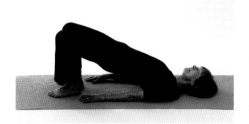

Hold for a moment and then release, rolling the spine back onto the floor. Take care to curl up and roll down. For a counter pose, hug the knees to the chest and rock from side to side.

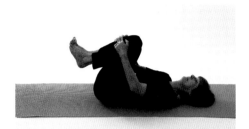

Finish all warm-up sequences by hugging the knees to the chest and rocking on the floor, giving the back a well-deserved massage.

5
HAND, SHOULDER AND NECK EXERCISES

Hand exercises

These exercises can be done kneeling, sitting or standing.

a)   Hold your arms out in front, make a fist with both hands then stretch the fingers out. Repeat several times.

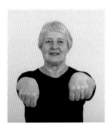
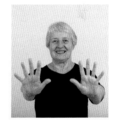

b)   Keep the arms out in front at shoulder height. Rotate the hands in opposite directions several times, then reverse the movement. Next, with the hands in a fist, on the downward movement rotate in the same fashion, and then spread the fingers out wide on the upward movement.

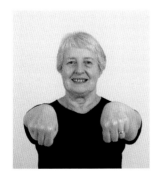
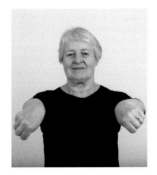
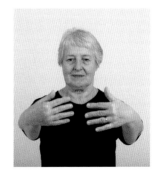

c) Place the hands on a firm surface, palms down. Gently put a little pressure on the hands, extending 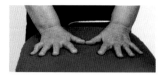 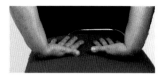 the wrists. Do the same with the back of the hands, applying a little pressure again. In older joints this can be painful so do not force it.

d) Place the palms on a firm surface and turn the hands so that the fingers are pointing back towards the body.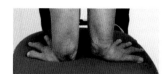

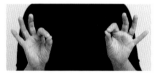 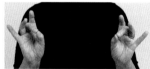 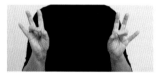

e) Try to touch each fingertip with the thumb.

f) Hold the thumb in the opposite hand. Take the hands away 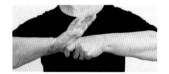 and up from the body. As you lower them pull the thumb very gently but firmly. Do this with each finger on both hands.

g) Place the fingers and thumb tips of both hands together and gently press the palms together, stretching the fingers slightly backwards.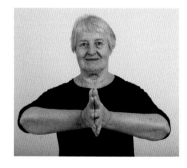

44

Shoulder exercises

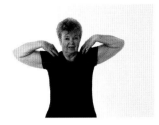

a)   Place the fingers on the shoulders and circle the arms forwards and

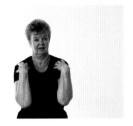

backwards six times in each direction.

b)   Take the arms out wide and straight at shoulder-height and make little circles with the arms, forwards and backwards, six times in each direction.

c)   Raise one arm above the head and bend it across the top of the head. Take the other hand to the elbow and gently pull the arm across the head. Repeat with the other arm.

d)   Using a strap take hold of each end, a little more than shoulder width apart. Raise the hands above the head and take them back as far as you can, keeping the arms straight. Lower the arms in front. Adjust the width of the strap for comfort if necessary.

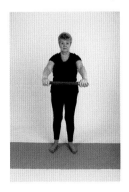
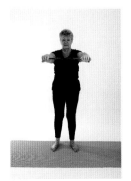
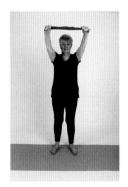

e) Stretch the arms out in front, then take them out wide and round to the back. Clasp the hands behind and lift the arms as high as possible, keeping

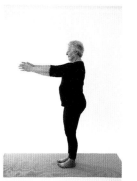 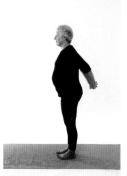

them straight. Hold for a moment and release, returning to the centre.

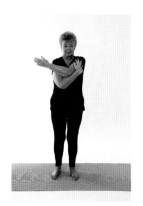 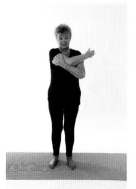

f) Bring an arm across the body and hug the upper part towards the chest. Repeat with the other arm.

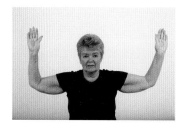

g) Raise the arms out to the side at shoulder height and bend the arms in front. Bring the arms

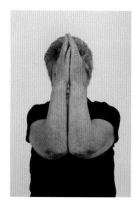

together in front of you, trying to touch elbows together, keeping the arms at shoulder height.

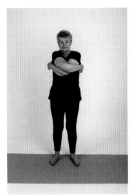
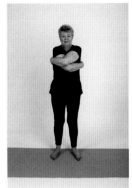

h) Give yourself a big hug, crossing the arms across the body. Then re-cross them with the other arm on top.

i) Rotate each arm slowly and mindfully, like a windmill going around.

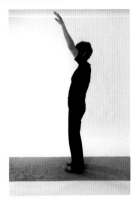
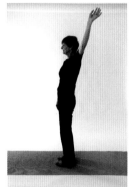

Repeat all these shoulder exercises several times.

Neck exercises

Sit comfortably, either on a chair or on the floor.

a) Take the chin to the chest. Gently roll the head round to the right shoulder, squeeze the head round a little more then release and roll the head down to the centre of the chest. Roll the head round to the other side, squeeze and roll back to the centre. Repeat three times to each side.

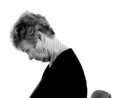
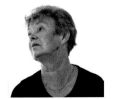
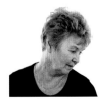

b)   Pretend the chin is resting on a table. Turn the head to the right, pause, then take it back to the centre. Turn the head to the left, pause and back to the centre again. Repeat three times.

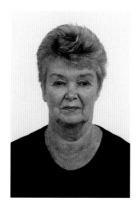 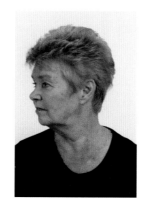 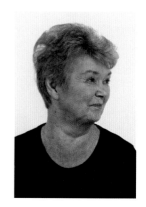

c)   Sitting up straight, keeping the neck long, take the right ear to the right shoulder, then back to the centre. Then take the ear over to the left shoulder and once again back to the centre. Repeat 3 times on each side.

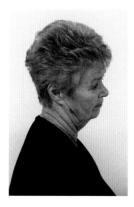 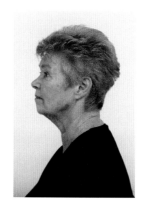 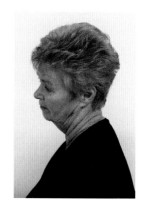

Try not to lift the shoulder, which would incorrectly bring towards the ear.

d)	Keeping the head upright, draw a figure of eight with the nose. From the centre take the nose up to the right, round and down and up to the centre, up to the left and down, back to the centre. Make the movement as big as possible.

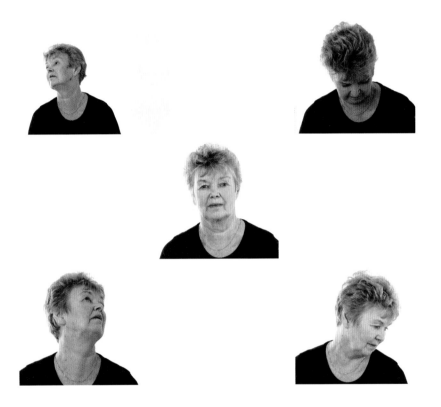

> **Always treat the neck very carefully, especially if you suffer from arthritis or any other neck problems.**

Take care of your body. It's the only place you have to live. Jim Rohn

6
EXERCISES AND STRETCHES

Hamstring stretch

Sit on a chair. Using a strap around the ball of the foot, bend and stretch the leg out as straight as possible. This can be done incorporating the breath: exhale on bending the leg,

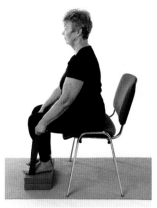 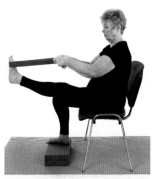

inhale as you stretch. Hold the stretch for a moment or two while also holding the breath. Return the leg to the starting position. Repeat with the other leg. Use a block under the feet if necessary.

Knee hugs

Sitting up straight on the chair, placing a block under the feet if necessary. Hug alternate knees to the chest.

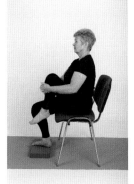 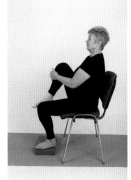

Hip circling

Stand by the chair, using it for stability if necessary. Circle the leg, making the movement as big as possible. Go to the other side and do the same. Repeat six times.

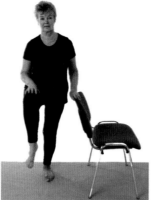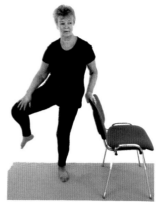

Dips

a)   With feet hip width apart, tuck your tail under, pull the abdomen in a little and keep the back straight to engage the pelvic floor muscles. Bend the knees as far as is comfortable and straighten. Repeat six times.

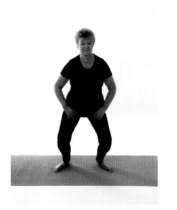

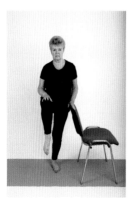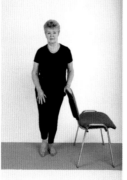

b)   Stand on the left leg, using a chair for balance if necessary. Bend the right leg up to a right angle. Lower it to the floor. Repeat 6 to 10 times. Change to the left leg and repeat.

c)   Keeping the knee bent, raise and lower it slightly, this time without the foot touching the floor. Repeat 6 to 10 times then change to the other leg.

Hip rolls

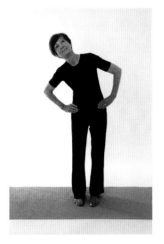

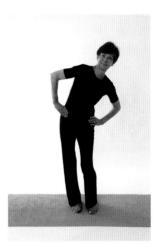

Stand tall with the hands on the hips. Tip the pelvis forward and back. Then tip the pelvis from side to side. Finally roll the hips in a circle, pushing forward, then to the side, then pushing backwards and finally to the other side. Do three or four rotations each way, very positively and slowly.

Standing tall (*tadasana*)

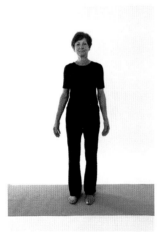

Tadasana is a pose for correct posture. Stand up straight, feet hip-width apart, being very aware of your body. Relax the shoulders, keep the neck long and the chin down. Tuck the tummy in hard and then relax slightly.

The knees should be straight but soft. Feel tall, close the eyes if you are happy to do so.

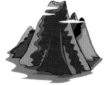

Breathe with a steady full breath. Feel the energy rise within you. You are a mountain. Stay for a while and then open the eyes and relax.

Leg lifts (standing)

Stand beside the chair, holding the back of it. Lift and straighten each leg in turn three to six times. Bend one leg at right angles in front of you and lift it up and as high as possible without losing your body alignment. Hold for a moment and lower. Repeat three to six times with each leg. Now raise the leg to the side, keeping the body 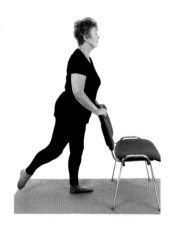 upright, without losing alignment. Hold and then lower. Repeat three to six times. Finally, stretch each leg out to the back the same number of times and then relax.

Leg swings

Using the chair for support allow each leg to swing loosely backwards and forwards about ten times.

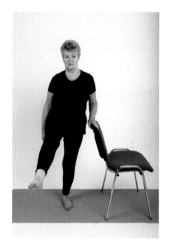 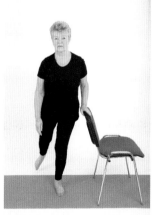

Standing balance and twist

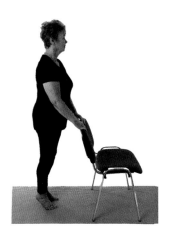

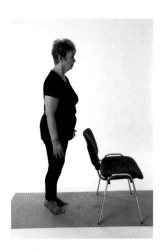

Using the chair for stability if necessary, rise up on tip-toe, hold the balance for a while, trying to let go of the chair if confident enough, then gently lower yourself. As your confidence improves (as it will), do this without the chair and twist round as far as possible to each side with the arms outstretched in front. Try this stretch first on flat feet then progress to tip toes.

Squats

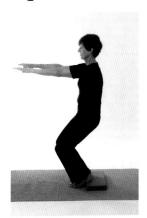

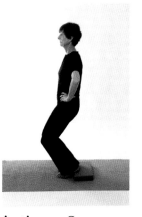

Stand with the feet 12 inches apart, feet facing forwards or slightly out to the sides. With a nice straight back place your hands on your waist (to start with) and squat as if sitting on a chair. Hold for a moment and then stand up again. Repeat six times. Once you gain strength raise your arms up to shoulder height as you squat and lower them as you stand up. Do not go so low that you cannot comfortably retrieve the posture. Use a chair for support if needed. It may be helpful to place a block under the heels.

Lightning bolt– a stronger squat.

Stand tall in *tadasana*, the mountain pose, the feet hip-width apart. Lift your arms up straight over your head and then bend the knees as if coming into a sitting position. Keep the back straight and the arms in line with the torso. Feel strong in this lightning shape. Do not bend so far that you cannot stand up again. Breathe deeply, then when ready stand up on an inhalation and lower the arms on the exhalation. Rest.

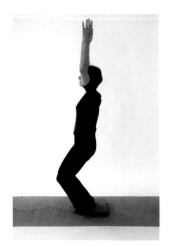

Side bend

Stand firmly with the feet hip-width apart. Hold the arms out loosely to the side. Keeping upright, raise one arm, stretch the body upwards and gently bend over to the side. Repeat three times to each side. This can also be done sitting on a chair with the legs together. Stretch to each side. Repeat again with both arms.

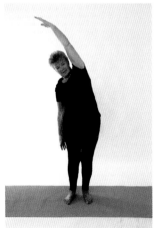
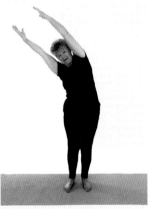

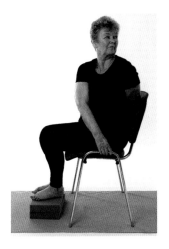

Twist on chair

Sit upright on a chair with the legs tightly together. Lift the torso and turn to the right as far as you can, reaching behind you to hold the back of the chair. Place the left hand on the outer side of the right thigh, helping to twist a little further. Hold and then release to the front. Do the same on the other side.

Tree

You may use a chair for support in this exercise if necessary. Stand in *tadasna*. Take the weight on to one leg and lift the other, placing it somewhere on the standing leg, avoiding the knee. Bring the hands

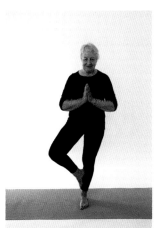
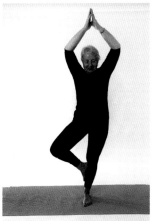
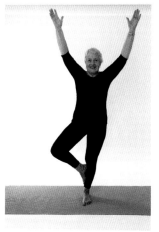

to *namaste*. Focus on a spot on the floor and slowly raise the arms above the head. Bring the hands together if possible. Hold for a few moments, breathing gently and steadily. Spread the arms to open 'branches' of your tree and then slowly lower them, taking the leg to the floor. Repeat on the other side. If using a chair, raise first one arm and then the other, letting go of the chair.

Modified Eagle

Stand in *tadasana*. Focus to restore your balance. Take the weight on one foot, spread the toes and when steady lift the foot and place on top of the other foot. Raise the arms above the head, cross them and place the palms together. Repeat on the other foot.

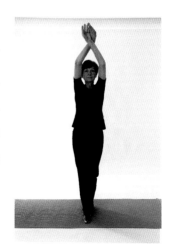

Seated forward bend

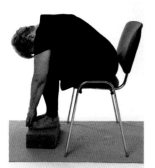

Sitting on a chair, part the legs to hip-width apart and bend forward. Alternatively sit with the legs together and bend forward over the knees. Try to relax the neck and shoulders and let the arms hang beside or in between your legs. Use a block under the feet if necessary.

Standing forward bend

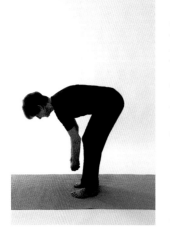

Stand with the feet hip-width apart, the knees soft. Slowly curl the spine down, then the shoulders, the chest, the waist and finally the hips. Relax the neck and shoulders and allow

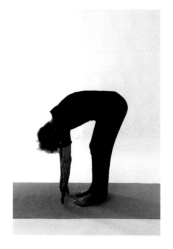

the body to hang. Retrieve the posture by bending the knees more, placing the hands on the thighs, bringing the head up, taking the bottom down and pushing up.

If you have high blood pressure or eye problems don't stay in the posture for too long – come straight out again.

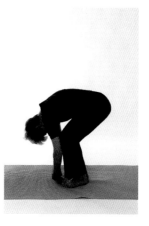

Back stretch

Stand behind the chair, two or three feet away. Bend forward to place your hands on the back of the chair, ideally at waist height, allowing the back to flatten. Straighten the legs as far as possible otherwise leave the knees slightly bent. Relax as much as possible. Wriggle the shoulders and try to relax the neck, bringing the head between the arms. To retrieve the posture step forward and push up on the chair.

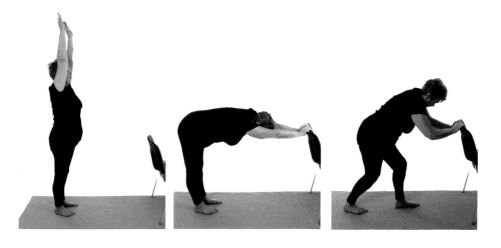

If this method is too strong, stand close to the chair and, keeping hold of it, walk back several steps until you are able to flatten your back. This way you avoid the strong forward bend. To retrieve the posture step forward and come up to standing, pushing up on the chair.

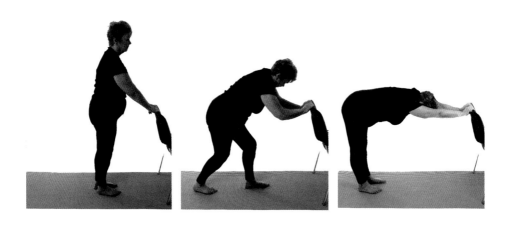

<u>Rear leg lift</u> – also known as The Warrior 3 posture.

Stand a couple of feet away from the chair. Lean forward, placing the hands on the back of the chair for support; then lift one leg up straight out at the back, making a 'T' shape with the body. This should tighten the muscles of the buttock. Lower the leg. Repeat two to three times each side. This can be tried without the chair when confidence allows.

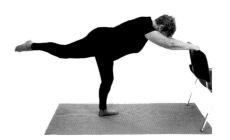

Flank stretch

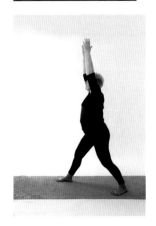

Come to a standing position, feet hip-width apart. Step forward with the right leg. Feel grounded and balanced. Stretch and raise the arms above the head. Fold forward to rest along the leg. Come to wherever you are comfortable. Try to relax in the forward bend and if possible bring the hands to the floor. To retrieve the posture bring the hands to the thigh and gently push up. Step the feet together and come to a standing position again. Do the same on the other side. Try to recover the posture in a neat and tidy fashion, with as much thought as possible. When strength allows, try lifting out of the posture with arms straight above the head.

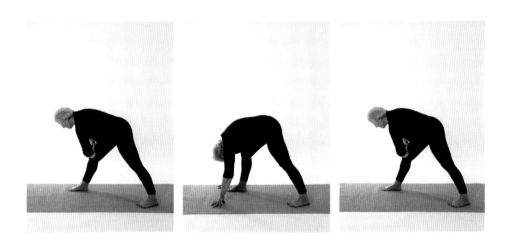

This can also be performed with the leg resting on the seat of a chair, first making sure that the chair is stable and doesn't move.

Combined flank and arm stretch

Stand tall. Step forward on the right leg. Feel grounded and balanced. Prepare the arms by clasping the hands behind the back. Fold forward as before, this time lifting the arms up behind you as well. Lower the arms, push the hands away towards the buttocks. Keeping the back straight, lift the head and come up to standing. Release the hands.

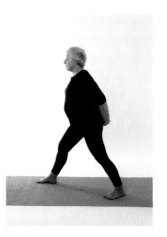

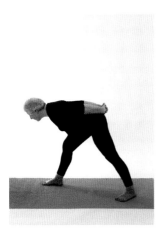 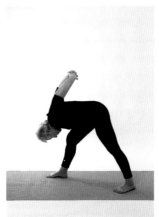

If there are problems with retrieving the posture in this way, release the hands first in order to place them on the thigh to push up.

7
POSTURES

Cat stretch – (on all fours)

This is not a traditional Yoga posture but a very beneficial stretch for the back.

Come onto the floor on hands and knees. The hands are shoulder-

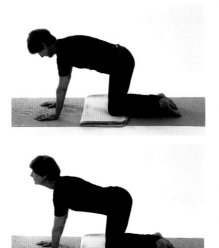

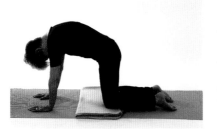

width apart and the knees hip-width apart. The spine is straight in a neutral position. On an inhalation allow the spine to extend, lifting the head and pushing the tail bone to the ceiling. On the exhalation raise the spine to curl upwards flexing it, lowering the head and tucking the tail under, stretching just like a cat.

Try to repeat this movement with the breath until it flows and then the eyes can be closed and focus can be brought to the movement. Take time to get the full stretch in each position, mentally following the curve of the spine in each direction.

An extra benefit can be achieved by stretching the leg out behind in a relaxed fashion and then, on the exhalation, curling the spine to bring the knee towards the forehead, touching it if possible.

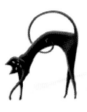

(See Chapter 3 for cat stretch in a sitting position.)

Balance in Cat

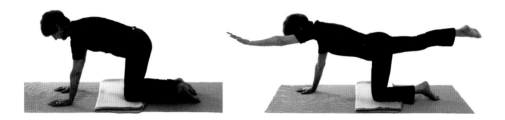

Still on all fours bring the knees closer together. Carefully finding the balance, raise the right leg and the left arm. Lower, do the same to the other side. It's easier if you take one limb away at a time rather than both together.

For something a little harder, try to raise the right arm and right leg. Hold and lower, then repeat to the left side.

Dog posture

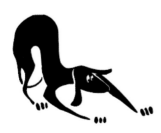

Come onto all fours on the floor with the knees hip-width apart. Spread your hands on the floor under the shoulders. Tuck the toes under, take the bottom back towards the heels, push into the heels and the knees

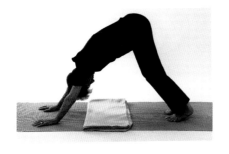

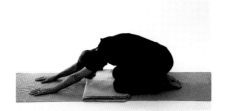

will lift. Push the buttocks up to the ceiling and stretch the back and shoulders out as much as possible. Relax the neck. Keep the knees soft but straighten the legs. Walk the feet on the spot giving each leg a gentle stretch. To retrieve, bend the knees to the floor taking the buttocks back onto the heels and rest in <u>swan</u> (see chapter 8).

Dog can also be attempted using a chair if using the floor is not for you.

Stand two or three feet away from the seat of the chair with feet hip-width apart. Hold the seat on either side and push the shoulders down and the buttocks up to the ceiling. Soften the knees if necessary and relax the

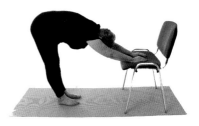

neck and shoulders. Hold for a second or two and then release back to standing.

Dog is an inverted posture and should not be attempted if you have eye problems or high blood pressure.

Cat and dog combination stretch

Start off in cat on all fours. Inhale; allow the spine to drop through, raising the head and pushing the tail up to the ceiling. Exhale; curling the spine,tucking the tail under and relaxing the neck

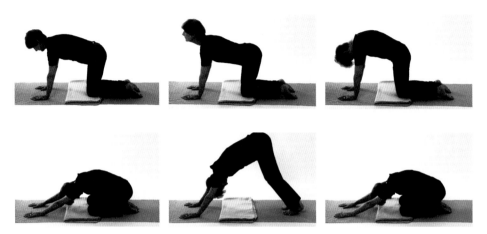

between the arms. Take the buttocks back toward the heels on the next inhalation. Tuck the toes under, push back into the feet and lift the knees.

Push up into dog position. Stretch in dog and then relax the knees back to the floor, unlock the toes and take the buttocks back to the heels, with the arms stretching away along the floor in front, into swan.

Bridge

This was included in the warm ups.

Lie on your back in semi-supine, feet hip-width apart, the arms loose and relaxed by your side. To start, tilt the pelvis by pushing the waist into the floor and curling the

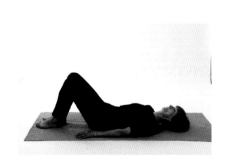

tailbone up without lifting off the floor. Next time do the same but go a little further and lift the buttocks off the floor.

Hold for a second or two, then roll back down onto the floor. Next time do the same but lift further if you can. Hold and then gently lower the body back onto the floor, vertebra by vertebra. Carry on in this way until you reach your maximum lift. Finally, hug the knees to the chest and then relax.

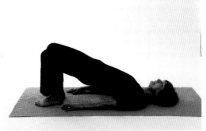

In this pose you can either inhale as you raise the body and exhale as you lower it or *vice versa,* whichever is more comfortable.

Alternate leg stretch

Sit on the floor, with the legs as wide apart as possible. A strap can be used around the foot to hold on to. Bend the left leg and bring the sole of the foot to the inside of the

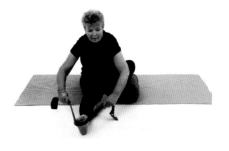

right thigh as far as possible, allowing the knee to drop out to the side. Support yourself on a block or padding if needed.

Turn to face down the right leg and, if using it, place the strap

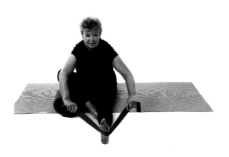

around the foot. Lift the body up straight and gently reach forward as far as you can. Keep the back straight, the head up and feel the stretch in the back of the leg. Do not compromise your posture by trying

67

to go too far and curling down to try to get the head on to the knees. Find your stretch and work gently with it.

To come back, drop the strap, take the hands to the floor and walk them up, raising the body. Repeat on the other side.

Triangle

Stand tall with the feet hip-width apart. Step forward on the right leg keeping as much width as possible (1 metre), turn the body towards the back leg, raise the arms to shoulder height. Tip the pelvis to the left and bend sideways towards the right leg, softening or bending the right knee if necessary. Try not to let the body bend forward; keep the alignment if possible. Do not over-bend and lose

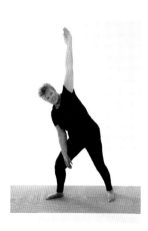

the dynamics of the posture. Hold, stretching the left arm up to the ceiling. Look straight ahead or to the ceiling, inhale and lift the body to the centre. Lower the arm, turn the body to the front and step forward. Repeat on the other side. This can be practiced against a wall to help to keep the alignment.

Warrior

Warrior pose is said to promote inner peace. It is also known as 'hero posture'. It builds strength and gives a feeling of wellbeing. There are three different versions of this posture.

Warrior 1

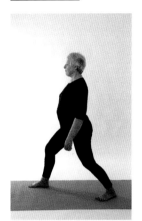

Stand straight and tall with the feet hip-width apart. Step forward with the right leg as far as is comfortable for you. Find your base by spreading the toes and feeling balanced. If necessary,

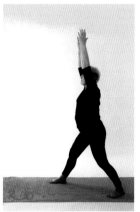

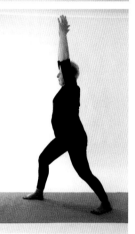

take the feet wider apart. It is now considered safer to keep the feet facing forward, lifting the back heel if necessary but keeping the back leg straight and strong. Technically, the front knee must not go over the front foot, but be kept at a right angle. Inhale and raise the arms over the head, stretching up. Exhale and bend the front knee. (Don't allow it to turn inwards.) Look straight ahead. Hold, relaxing the shoulders and trying to keep the body upright. Keep breathing while you hold. Inhale, straighten the knee then exhale and lower the arms to the side. Step both feet together. Relax and experience how the body feels. Repeat on the other side.

Warrior 2

Stand straight. Step forward exactly as before onto the right leg, keeping as much width as possible. Spread the toes and feel stable and grounded. Inhale, raising the arms overhead, as in Warrior 1. Exhale and bend the knee as before. Keep the body as upright as

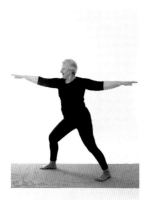

possible. Keep breathing steadily and open the arms to shoulder height. Keep facing forwards. Feel strong. Hold for a little while, then bring the arms up overhead again. On an inhalation straighten the leg and exhale, lowering the arms and stepping forward. Repeat on the other side.

Warrior 3

Prepare as for warrior 1 with the arms above the head. Take the weight onto the right leg. Feel balanced. Now take the body into a forward table top bend or right angle. Raise the left leg so that the body is in a 'T' shape. This is a more advanced posture needing strength and confidence so it is advisable to use a chair for balance until you feel confident. Repeat with the other leg.

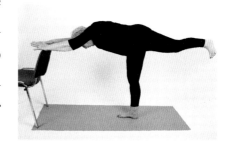

Sphinx and modified Cobra

Lie on your front on the floor. Take the feet hip-width apart. Stretch the arms out in front on the floor. The forehead rests on the floor. Inhale and exhale, walk the hands in towards the body one span at a time. Do this until the elbows are under the shoulders. Lift the head, lengthen the neck, drop the shoulders

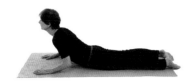

and breathe steadily. Pushing the pubic bone down into the floor, take your awareness into the spine. Hold and when ready, walk the hands away and lower the body down. Bring the arms beside the body and rest with the head to one side. Repeat two to four times. Take the head to the opposite side each time.

Lie on the floor as before, the forehead resting on the floor. Bring the hands level with the eyes. Gently raise the head and then the shoulders off the floor. Lengthen the neck, drop the shoulders and try to relax the upper body. Push the pubic bone into the floor. Breathe and hold, then slowly lower the body back to the floor. Relax with the head on one side and the arms to the sides. For a counter pose take the hands back under the shoulders and push the body back into swan.

Locust

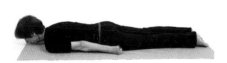 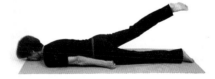

Lie on your front on the floor, feet together, resting the chin on the floor. Place your fists, thumbs down, firmly against the floor at the side of your body. Push against the floor with the fists and raise the right leg as high as possible. Hold and then lower. Repeat, raising the left leg. Relax.

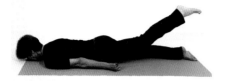 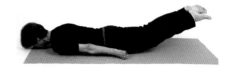

Now repeat the same procedure but this time raise both legs. This might be impossible but attempt the posture even though the feet may not leave the floor. You are still doing the work. Relax.

Always remember that if you have worked strenuously you need to rest between postures and allow the breath to settle.

8

SOME RELAXING POSTURES

Swan

Swan is a relaxing position to use between postures. Kneel on the floor with the toes not tucked under. Take the buttocks back onto

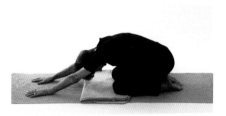

the heels as far as possible. Stretch the arms out in front along the floor, bringing the forehead towards the floor as far as possible. You can support the head on fists or a block if you wish or just allow the neck and head to relax without support.

Child pose

Another relaxing posture if you are able to come down onto the floor. Kneel, bending the body forwards over the thighs with the arms

beside the body. This is not for everyone especially if the head does not reach the floor or you don't like feeling constricted around the abdomen. A block can be used to support the forehead.

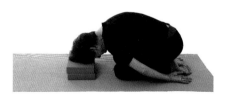

You could also sit on a chair and allow the body to relax over the legs with the arms hanging to the side.

Hare pose

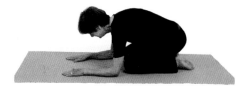

This is similar to the child pose but kneeling low and resting the abdomen on the thighs, facing forwards with the forearms on the floor. This is a better posture if you suffer from eye problems or high blood pressure or don't feel comfortable with being too low and feeling constricted.

Semi-supine

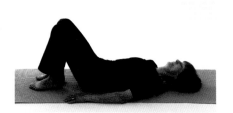

Lie on your back with the knees bent, the arms away from the body and the spine pressed into the floor. Relax the face and shoulders, breathe steadily and rest.

Feet and legs in the air

(an inverted posture)

I have not taught the shoulder stand in this manual because if you are new to Yoga practice and of a certain age I do not think it

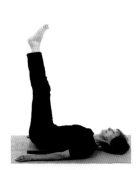

advisable to start. However it is nice to lie on the floor with a block under the buttocks and place the feet and legs up against a wall. You can also push against the wall with the feet and lift the buttocks off the floor a few inches. You can also place the legs on the seat of a chair or just rest with the legs in the air unsupported.

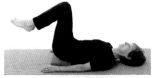

Corpse

Lie on your back with the legs out straight. The head should be central, resting comfortably on the floor or a block, blanket or cushion. The arms are away from the body at the side and the legs wider than hip-width apart.

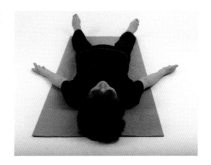

Relax the face, shoulders, arms and legs. Allow the breathing to settle and rest.

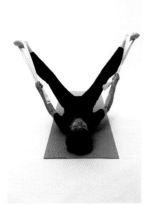

Legs wide apart in the air – using straps

This posture looks very undignified and strange but it is exceedingly comfortable and relaxing.

All these positions are very good for varicose veins and very refreshing for the legs in general.

***The more man meditates upon good thoughts
the better will be his world and the world
at large.*** Confucius

9
MEDITATION

Theoretically, the practice of meditation is intended to withdraw the personal mind from its persistent preoccupation with worldly affairs and to train it to concern itself with matters that lead to the understanding of spiritual realities.

Adelaide Gardener

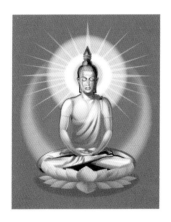

<u>Why meditate?</u>

Caroline Myss suggests:-

a)   To keep ourselves centred when all around us is chaos.

b)   <u>Not</u> to find eternal happiness, but to cultivate an abiding calmness to help us cope with whatever life throws at us. Our journey through life is a learning curve, good or bad. It's the dark times that help us to see God.

c)   To find the light. We have to enter the darkness in order to see the light.

d)   To help us find God (whatever our concept is of God) in our ordinary lives without the necessity of a monastic calling.

A lot of people think of meditation as being something mysterious and difficult, needing very serious training. This is not the case. It does however need discipline and commitment to regular practice. Nowadays we are turning more and more to this practice in order to relieve the stresses of a frantic, noisy, modern life. Science and the medical profession have begun to realise that meditation does have a beneficial effect on the mind-body connection, and that a quiet relaxed mind brings about the same effect on the body.

It is difficult to describe exactly what happens during meditation. It needs to be experienced rather than described. There are many methods that can be used in order to calm the mind. You need to find the one that suits you best.

The four main requirements

1)   A quiet place

It is difficult to meditate in a place that is noisy or where there aredistractions. Try to make a place in your home specifically for meditation. If space is limited have a corner of the room with perhaps a special chair or a table with some flowers and a picture of your favourite spiritual icon on it. Make yourself comfortable, turn off the telephone and tell other members of the house that you require some quiet undisturbed time. If you have a room to go to have a polite 'Do Not Disturb' sign on the door. If you are using music put it on very quietly; light a candle if you wish to set the scene.

2)   <u>A comfortable, warm position</u>

If there is discomfort or pain it will be impossible to settle.

Have a special blanket to wrap around you if chilly.

3)   <u>A passive attitude</u>

You should let go of the expectation of 'result'. No two experiences of meditation will ever be the same.

4)   <u>A mental device</u>

Have something on which to focus and concentrate the mind to exclude distractions. In Yoga we use sight, sound and breath. The sound can be quiet, soothing music. For sight we can gaze at a candle, a crystal or a picture and for breath there are many different breathing techniques.

A very simple Yogic breath:

Make yourself comfortable and try to relax any tension in the neck and shoulders. Close the eyes or just lower and soften the gaze. Take two or three deep breaths in through the nose and out through the mouth, mentally letting go if possible. Now let the breath settle but stay with it, noting the passage of air through the nose and down to the lungs. Be aware of the movement of the rib cage and the passage of air out through the nose. Do this for several minutes then let it go and sit very still; every time the mind wanders gently bring it back to focus on the breath, the tip of the nose or the music, or gaze at the candle for a while before closing the eyes again.

To start with, set a short time for meditation – 5 minutes, no more – until you begin to feel comfortable with the practice. Then you can lengthen it gradually.

Just remember that when you have mastered the knack of switching off and just being quiet within yourself, you will be able to meditate anywhere and at any time. It's not the rocket science that some would have you believe.

BIBLIOGRAPHY AND OTHER SOURCES

Reiki and the Seven Chakras Richard Ellis. ISBN 978 0 091 88290 7

The Science of Yoga Swami Savananda.

Yoga for Real Life Maya Fiennes. ISBN 978 1 84354 937 6

Yoga 28 day Exercise Plan Richard Hittleman. ISBN 0 600 39508 1

Easy does it Yoga Alice Christensen & David Rankin.
 ISBN 0 06 2501453

The Complete Idiots Guide to Yoga (second edition) Joan Budilovsky
    and Eve Adamson. ISBN 0 02 863970 7

British Wheel Of Yoga handouts.

Notes From my Yoga teacher – Vonnie Bloom.

Meditation Notes, with acknowledgement to John Cain's web site.

Meditation Notes from my tutor Megan Joyce.

Audio Collection Caroline Myss Ph.D.

How to use YOGA Mira Mehta. ISBN 1 84309 780 X

Hatha Yoga Pradipika Swami Muktibodhananda.
   ISBN 81 85787 38 7

Yoga for Body Breath and Mind A. G Mohan. ISBN 1 57062 977 3

The Complete Book of Yoga Sri Ananda. ISBN 81 222 0094 X

The Beginners Guide to Classic Yoga Frances Houlahan. ISBN 1
    85605692 9

Di Kendal – Study Day Notes

Acknowledgements

Many thanks go to Vonnie Bloom, Dee Rhodes, Lesley & Cris and my family for their help and support. Thanks also to Mandy-Lee Mouncer (mandymouncer@gmail.com) for her photographic skills. Thanks also to Sacred Centers, Anodea Judith and the website WWW.SacredCenters.com for *chakra* information and illustrations. All the models are in their seventies and all suffer from the usual age-related problems.

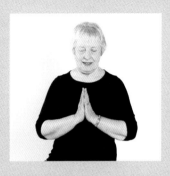

The practice of Yoga is a personal journey
without a goal or the need to achieve,
which will lead you to a place of contentment,
liberation and peace.

OM SHANTI, SHANTI, SHANTI

MY PROGRESS DIARY

_____

_____

_____

_____

_____

_____

_____

_____

_____

_____

_____

_____

_____

_____

_____

_____

_____

_____

_____

_____

_____

_____

_____

_____

MY PROGRESS DIARY

_____

_____

_____

_____

_____

_____

_____

_____

_____

_____

_____

_____

_____

_____

_____

_____

_____

_____

_____

_____

_____

_____

_____

_____

_____

MY PROGRESS DIARY

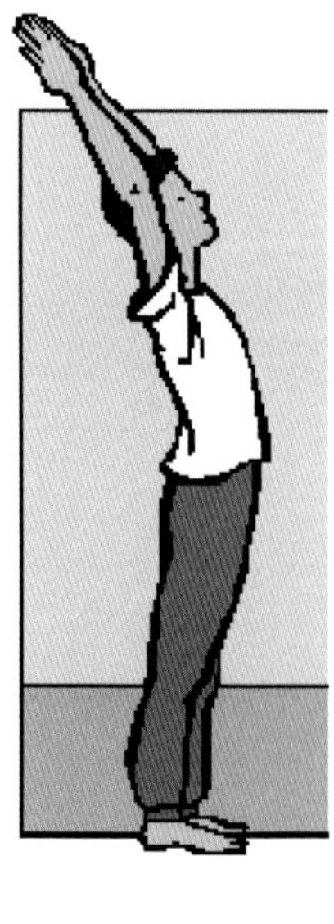

_____

_____

_____

_____

_____

_____

_____

_____

_____

_____

_____

_____

_____

_____

_____

_____

_____

_____

_____

_____

_____

_____

_____

_____

MY PROGRESS DIARY

MY PROGRESS DIARY